Frenching Your Food

7 Guilt-Free French Diet Tips
to Slim Down, Look Younger and
Live Longer without Calorie-Counting
or Strenuous Exercise

Adrienne N. Hew, C.N.
The Nutrition Heretic

EDITED BY LAUREN TEDROW

ISBN: 1495939022
ISBN-13: 978-1495939020

Disclaimer

The content of this book is provided as information only and may not be construed as medical or health advice. No action or inaction should be taken solely on the basis of the information provided here. Please consult with a licensed health professional or doctor on any matter relating to your health and wellbeing.

The information and opinions expressed in this book are believed to be accurate and factual based upon the resources available to the authors at the time of writing. Readers who fail to consult with the appropriate health authorities assume the risk of any and all injuries.

The publisher is not responsible for errors or omissions.

DEDICATION

To the countless French women,
who have taught me how to French

"Whenever you find yourself on the side of the majority, it is time to pause and reflect."

- Mark Twain

Table of Contents

Pucker Up

Frenching food is an art that Americans have been enthralled with for decades. Study after study has proven that the French diet has helped French people to attain longer, happier, and thinner lives. Sadly, when we Americans open our mouths to eat, we do so with an aggression and disdain for food that the French find rather *gauche*, vulgar and uncivilized. No matter what truths we learn about the French diet, we continue to hold strong to our bland and guilt-filled food attitudes while expecting a daily glass of red wine to make up for any shortcomings.

Seduced by the fallacies invented and perpetuated by the Big Health Food industry (the little brother of Big Agriculture and Big Pharma), it would appear that the French defy all laws of nature. They supposedly eat "all the wrong things" such as plenty of pork, eggs, butter, cream and other foods that are high in fat and cholesterol, yet they are far healthier than us. Since "everybody knows" that fat and cholesterol are a no-no for good health, assessments of the healthy French diet come with warnings to replace all fat and cholesterol-containing foods with synthetic, processed food replacements.

As a compromise, the genius scientists working for Big Health Food have determined that red wine somehow miraculously patches the "flaws" in the French diet. Yes, it seems that no matter how badly we eat, even if we eat fat -- which of course we do not because we are smart enough not to -- red wine will solve all of our health problems, while we lose weight and live longer. So what is the final result of all this scientific wisdom? We have become a nation of winos, obsessed with ultra-low fat dieting, who gorge ourselves highly processed diets that fit the "perfect diet" laid out by paid-for science.

This mindset has paved the way for a plethora of acceptable eating disorders that conveniently fit into what Big Health Food and its older siblings want us to believe. Raw food, vegan, fruitarian, breatharian and to some extent Paleolithic and macrobiotic diets are such diets that play into the hands of Big Health Food. Most people think of these diets as more natural than the Standard Modern Diet, but in fact, very often many of them -- especially from the vegetarian side of the spectrum -- are just as bad, if not worse. Most soy products; dairy, meat and egg substitutes; hemp; agave; gluten-free foods; and canola oil are just a small sampling of popular "health foods" that rake in billions of dollars annually for food processing companies at the expense of our health.

These so-called health foods have virtually taken over the American table for one very important reason: the stringent dietary guidelines set up for us by Big Health Food are virtually impossible to achieve in nature. Some experts tell us to eliminate all fat, salt, and protein, sucking all of the gratification and nutritional value out of our meals (yes, fat, salt and protein are crucial to good health). Others want us to eliminate most sugars (to some extent, I actually agree with this point of view). Unfortunately, most from the latter group suggest replacing sugar with loads of fruit sweeteners, chemical-based substitutes and highly processed replacements like agave syrup. Most every one of these meat, fat, salt and sugar substitutes that I can think of has been shown to carry with it a new crop of rare diseases, allergies, addictions, and in many cases, weight gain.

Interestingly enough, the French have, for the most part, kept many of these fake health foods at bay. Yet as more French people take up residence in the United States, Britain and other

English-speaking countries, their food habits are becoming clouded by the desire to conform to the "smart" way of eating.

A good example of this is shown in Mireille Guiliano's popular book, *French Women Don't Get Fat*. Overall, I felt that the book was excellent. However, given my more than 25 years of experience eating with French women, I could not help, but see a rather large discrepancy between Guiliano's current perspective on food and what I have learned from all other French women in years past. It seems that Guiliano now Frenches like an American.

Unlike so many books about health and weight loss, *French Women Don't Get Fat* concerns itself relatively little with the typical mathematical equation of calories in, calories out that features so prominently in most American weight loss books. Instead, Guiliano focuses more on the preservatives and on the *most* processed garbage that many Americans don't think twice about putting in their mouths. This is a major triumph that nutrition gurus in this country need to start recognizing and teaching.

However, the book actually features relatively few stories of how Guiliano herself controls her weight. Many of her anecdotes are about Americans to whom she has given a couple of diet tips or her aunt who introduced her to a near-starvation method of quickly shedding water weight over the weekend. Given the fact that so many Americans—including the ones whom she has coached—eat a steady diet of items poured from cardboard boxes, it is easy to see why these people successfully shed the pounds by following her core method of actually eating foods found in nature. And of course, eating little more than puréed leek soup for 48 hours is bound to draw excess fluids from most anybody who does not have a metabolic issue.

Overall, Guiliano and I differ little in our opinions on food, however, in some places her commentary reminds me of the new food attitudes that I am beginning to see in a few of my French friends (and friends from other parts of the world) who either moved to the U.S., married an American or hang out in health food stores, which are largely, although not completely, influenced by American trends.

Many of these people had never even heard of concepts such as super low fat diets or getting protein from anything other than an animal product 20 to 25 years ago when I was a believer in such things. However, with globalization and the Internet, this "new wisdom" is gaining acceptance in France as it is in other countries once known for their impressive lifespans and waistlines. And just as in the United States, their lives are being cut short by disease as their waistlines expand after implementing new diet trends that are designed to boost corporate profits over human health.

While Guiliano does an excellent job of emphasizing certain real foods that most Americans fear, as I read more closely, I realized that she left out one very important aspect of the French diet – the difference between how the French and Americans relate to food. Yes, she discusses how the French love to talk about and prepare delicious meals even before the current meal is done, but she stops just short of looking at the broken relationship that the average American has for food. That is what this book will attempt to shed light on.

Before moving forward, let's get one thing clear. I am not a psychologist. So while this book is largely a discussion on the psychology of nutrition, it is coming from the experience of a nutritionist.

It wasn't until after graduation when I began practicing nutrition that I realized just how many psychological issues needed to be addressed to help people make the best choices for themselves. No matter how much people claimed to want to be healthy, what they really wanted was sexy talk with a lot of hype or even blatant lies about miraculous, even unrealistic weight loss goals.

Here I was teaching people how to feel confident eating the delicious foods of their ancestors – often foods they remembered fondly from their childhood and was meeting with an unexplainable resistance and guilt by my clients. In those early days, many of them were turning follow people advocating super-restrictive diets such as vegetarian, macrobiotic or vegan diets that made them sick and gain weight.

On the far end of the spectrum, I had people participating in or seriously contemplating even more disturbing cult-like rituals of consuming their own urine and excrement. That was the last straw! "Really? You'd rather eat a steady diet of feces instead of butter?" was all I could think. It became clear to me that as a people, our relationship with food had become so strained that we no longer trusted food. We had now reached a point where we were willing to trust *anything else* instead. To this day, we are still looking for love in all the wrong places and we are paying a high price for it with our health and mental wellbeing.

Selling empty promises was, and still is, difficult for me to do. I find it disingenuous as a health professional to perpetuate the lies of Big Health Food, Big Ag, Big Pharma, the American Dietetics Association and 99% of the health gurus in the Western Hemisphere at the expense of an individual's health for profit. That is why I had to write this book.

In this book, I will reveal valuable health tips that I have learned over the years from the *healthy*, and consequently, thin French women that I have known. The ones who are thin (or fat) and *unhealthy* <u>don't</u> follow this advice.

For years, I did not follow this advice either. Despite the fact that I could see the evidence of the diet working for these women and having learned for so long that the French held the keys to good health, I could not reconcile what I was seeing with my eyes with the so-called science that I had learned in school and in trendy health magazines. Only later did I realize that these resources gave their own misguided spin on what constituted the healthy French diet. Like so many, I chose to follow the self-loathing approach endorsed by American scientists, the American Dietetic Association and the American Medical Association—and that advice nearly killed me.

This book is not so much about the "best" and "worst" foods to eat. It is about how the French (and in particular skinny French women) bring sensuality and carnal pleasure to the table. It is about how American women who struggle to lose weight can bring that same self-nurturing element to their food experience. As such, the discussion does not cover things like the virtues of organics or the hazards of nitrates in cured meats like ham and sausage. Rather it is a celebration of food, of life, and of you.

Learning to Open Wide

I was rather ashamed at the time, but now I am proud to say that a 70-year old woman was the first person to teach me how to French. I remember staring into her bright grey eyes across the table of a dimly lit kitchen as she attempted to romance me with tales of the French way to eat. As sweet as they were, her words were wasted on me for many long and painful years.

Modernity was the name of my game. I had just turned 18 and was looking for the latest thrill in food trends, not the traditional, respectful relationship of every generation that preceded mine.

As a child of the 70s, I allowed myself to be wooed by every new food "improvement" that lined store shelves. Left behind were a string of addictions (primarily to sugar), broken promises and lowered self-esteem. It would be another seven years before I would open my eyes wide enough to decide to leave this abusive relationship for good.

Looking back on my early health history, I had always thought that my body was cursed at conception. Seasonal battles with eczema and chronic ear infections plagued me. Gradually, the ear infections gave way to frequent nosebleeds. Eventually the nosebleeds made room for asthma, acne, a pre-cancerous cervical condition and ovarian cysts. Through it all, the one thing that never plagued me was my weight... Until I tried to lose a few pounds.

Why, oh why do young women succumb to social pressures that lead to low self-esteem and all the unwise decisions that stem from it? Wearing a size six or eight was not good enough for me when other women my age were wearing size two or even zero. It was precisely this unreasonable expectation that sent me looking for food's affections in all the wrong places. Whether my reasons for wanting to shed a few pounds were justified or not, it was the start of my weight loss battle as well as the catalyst that took my already poor health to its lowest point.

When I had moved to France, I thought that I already knew how to French. After all, I had already spent a decade dedicating much of my waking hours to both the language and culture.

Then the American Dietetic Association (ADA) distracted my attention, touting the virtues of a low-fat, grain-based *vegetarianesque* diet. It was hard to reconcile the old-fashioned French diet with all its butter and cheese and this new and exciting diet, which was "supported by the best science in the world", but I eventually gave myself over to this new bad boy on the block.

This boy lied to me – repeatedly. The biggest lie he told me was that Frenching involved a paradox where the consumption of red wine would magically undo the supposed damage caused by all the fat the French ate. Yet he still cautioned me to avoid as much of the fat, dairy and meat the French ate as possible.

Suffice it to say that he was not a good influence on me. I allowed him to seduce me with promises of thinness and vibrant health. And when he didn't deliver on those promises, I began to hate my body so much that I spent weeks at a time cursing food and even starving myself until my head would begin to pound from the nutrient deprivation. It was always my fault – my body's fault, not his.

The family I lived with in France was of Italian origin. They embraced the type of diet that the ADA wanted me on: Lots of bread, potatoes, beans, and other starches; some salads; olive oil; and relatively small amounts meat. You would think that since three of the four family members were obese, I would have stopped to consider *this* paradox. But I did not. I simply assumed that they consumed far too many calories. It is entirely probable that they did eat too much in general as excessive carbohydrate consumption leads to uncontrolled appetite for many people, but I later learned that eating so many carbohydrates even without the increase in appetite leads to obesity for most people as well.

When Madame Claudine, our 70-year old neighbor, walked in one day with her charming sweet talk about how she could teach me to French, I was repulsed. I was convinced that she was some dirty old woman looking for a thrill at the expense of some naïve college students. Looking back, however, I now recognize Claudine's true beauty. She was not super-skinny, but she was far from being fat. Although she was in her 70s, her soft barely wrinkled skin did not show her chronological age. Her advice was not ego-driven as it is for so many others who try to sweet talk us with dietary promises. It came from the heart. It was an attempt to pass the torch of knowledge gathered from life experience.

Oh, how I wish I had not been so stubborn! I would have saved myself so many weight and health problems. While I was eating the "healthy" diet of my obese host family, I was rejecting the wisdom of this healthy woman of normal size. How ludicrous is that?

I never gained a ton of weight living in that jumbo-sized household, nor did I ever tip the scales at more than maybe 130 lbs. during that year. I did, however, begin to pack on some extra pudginess around the middle despite my one-and-a-half to three-hour brisk walks to and from school each day. Today, I have no doubt that if I followed the advice of my French neighbor, I would have lost 5 lbs. or more instead of gaining them.

Still wanting to earn the undying love of my bad-boy diet, upon my return to the U.S., I made a commitment to turn my life over to a diet that was even lower in fat, meat, dairy and calories. I dove head first into an organic, health food store lifestyle. Meat, dairy and fat were condiments—if ever eaten at all—as I dramatically increased my raw vegetable consumption.

During that time, I began working for a French newspaper in New York City. The French women I worked with introduced me to even more Frenching techniques that I just could not fathom. As with Claudine, I thought they were behind the times. And even though most of them were slimmer than me, I thought that what they were saying would not work *for me* even though I refused to try it. That is not to say that we did not enjoy some nice meals together in good French restaurants from time to time. I was not *that* much of a fanatic. However, when I did, I felt like I had cheated on my diet and had to scrub the taste of dairy, meat and fat from my mouth.

Two years later, shortly after leaving the newspaper, I was diagnosed with cervical dysplasia (a pre-cancerous condition) and ovarian cysts. It took several years before I learned that my vulgar, Americanized attempt at Frenching had such a strong correlation with such conditions. Like so many in that position, I chalked it up to a polluted *outer* environment and heredity (even though I was the first person in my family to suffer from any of these problems).

A few years later, I put on about 20 lbs. virtually overnight and seemingly for no reason. Along with the weight gain came lethargy (chronic fatigue syndrome), cracked and bleeding eczema that was now year round, yeast syndrome, and hypothyroidism. I was miserable, sick and on the verge of suicide. My bad boy diet abused me, then abandoned me and left me for dead.

In 1995, I learned from a highly skilled doctor that it was not only OK, but imperative that I begin Frenching Claudine's way. It was precisely at the moment that I began to fully give myself over to the inner most desires of my body that my health began to turn around. Instead of watching my body deteriorate further as had happened when I was under the spell of the ADA's healthy diet, within 2 months I dropped the 20 lbs I had struggled to let go of for the previous few years. Simultaneously, I experienced increased energy, clear skin for the first time in my life and improved digestion.

The funny part is that as my doctor was telling me what to

eat to get well, I thought to myself "I knew it!" Not with the same smug conviction I had when I was ignoring the words of wise French women, but for the first time I had a health *authority* giving me <u>permission</u> to eat in a way that supported what these women had been telling me. Unlike most doctors, this doctor had a strong background in nutrition. Previously, even though I had rejected the information I had learned from skinny French women, there was part of me that recognized that we humans did not get to the modern era on a diet of soy burgers and fake milk. While a part of me wanted to believe them, I was too self-righteous to give any credence to their intelligence even though they were living proof of a diet that kept them slim, living long and looking great as they aged.

Sadly, I see many people (clients, friends, and family) go down this road today. As was once my case, their level of education will not allow them to accept the truth despite mountains of evidence. The result is damaged digestion, rampant allergies, gluten intolerance, skin conditions, infertility, autism and in many cases cancer.

This phenomenon does not seem to be slowing down either. Over and over again, I talk to Americans who visit other countries like Japan, China, France, Italy, or Greece and talk about how they spent their entire visit dodging certain foods because they were "fattening" or "unhealthy". This is NEVER from experience, but simply because of their preconceived notions. Often, they tack on a story about how they had to educate their hosts in a foreign land about health even though their hosts were way healthier than them!

One main distinction between their situations and my

previous one is that these people are more likely to shun the advice of a licensed health practitioner with a good track record. Instead they choose to hand authority over to a friend, celebrity or a doctor with NO nutritional training who tells them the same kind of broken advice they learned on the evening news. Remind you of someone?

It is easy for me to spot this dysfunction because, as stated before, I did something very similar at one time. On more than one occasion, I had been known to tell healthy people that they knew nothing about "modern health", while my body was clearly suffering from the benefit of my supposed wisdom. It was as if I believed on some level that modern humans had different nutritional requirements than our ancient ancestors and even as recent as my grandparents. If I had listened sooner to many of these tips, I would have saved myself a lot of pain, suffering and MONEY! Hopefully sharing this French health wisdom will help to free you from your nutritional prejudices so that you too can give yourself over to the pleasures of the French table.

Tip #1: Linguistic Lobsters

Americans wrestle with the concept of protein. Back in the 1980s, we began buying into the idea of beans providing an adequate supply. Today, we have succumbed to even more ridiculous claims of everything from nuts and seeds to fruits and green leafy vegetables providing adequate protein. This myth has had a disastrous effect on our waistlines and our overall health.

When I worked for the French-American newspaper in New York, there was always talk of diets and dieting. Even the skinniest of my colleagues was always talking about some diet or other.

Like so many people moving to the United States, they found their weight creep up after a few months of arriving and suddenly had to actively work to keep the numbers on the scale from rising.

It did not take me long to join in with the fun. Along with the others, I tried different fads (like restricting calories to 1000 per day for three days and then eating anything I wanted for the other four days of the week) and skipping breakfast, but when these women told me that beans were fattening, I begged to differ. How could beans be fattening, I wondered, when they don't even contain any fat?

Unfortunately, I did not even attempt to educate myself (perhaps if the Internet were readily available at that time I would have). Instead, I wrote them off as a bunch of misinformed rubes, who were behind the times. How obnoxious is that???

At the time, I believed the hype that beans were going to save the planet by reducing the need for animal foods. They were considered a form of zero fat protein, after all, weren't they?

Not to these French women! When they wanted protein, they ate protein. In other words, COMPLETE protein in the form of animal products like meat (including beef, pork, lamb, chicken, fish, seafood), organ meats, eggs and dairy. They understood that the body would not settle for less.

When I began actually studying nutrition in a scholastic setting, I realized just how faulty it was to believe that beans or nuts are a source of protein. These foods contain amino acids, which are the building blocks of protein, but the plant world does not supply any food that is a complete source of *all* the amino acids necessary to make even one unit of complete protein -- no matter what companies that make meat replacement products tell you.

And if you have bought into the idea that combining beans with a grain like rice or bread will make up the balance, it is time to reevaluate this information too. Trying to figure out which grain would supply the right amounts of the missing amino acid in your beans to create a complete protein is somewhat akin to playing Russian roulette. It is not hard to lose this guessing game and the results can be disastrous.

Even in carefully controlled diets, the human body is ill-suited to digesting cellulose (the wall protecting the nutrients in plants) and therefore cannot liberate the amino acids within.

In the absence of animal-based foods at the same meal and without cooking, humans have an even more difficult time converting amino acids into protein. This makes complete sense to me now as I look at traditional diets where rice and beans, for example, are consumed with pieces of pork, pork fat, chicken stock, fish or dairy. Another good example is miso soup. According to my Japanese (not Japanese-American) friends and my extensive collection of authentic Japanese cookbooks, it is typically made from a fish broth base (*dashi*) and followed by a meal that contains pork, fish or some other form of animal protein.

This book, however, is about the French diet and the French women in my office warned me how difficult it was to digest beans and how even when properly prepared (pre-soaked and rinsed before cooking) could easily lead to bloating and abdominal distention. They also recognized them as fattening because of their carbohydrate load (something else I found ridiculous at the time). I wish I had listened because my high bean diet led to serious digestive damage within a few years. The effect was so bad that it took many years before I could digest them adequately again.

Now I can eat beans and still enjoy them from time to time, but I understand that they are not a cure for anything and merely a nice occasional compliment to an already nutritious meal. I still tread carefully as I do not want my health to end up where it was at the height of my digestive troubles.

It is a disturbing trend that more and more people are not modeling the success of the French, but instead are opting for politically correct trends based upon wishful thinking and slick marketing. Sausages and hot dogs are out because of the perception that they contain toxin-filled organ meats. The French, on the other hand, know that organ meats are the most nourishing part of the animal. Beef is shunned in favor of chicken because red meat is "bad," yet the French know that beef (especially pastured beef) is a powerhouse of nutrients that builds blood, aids in weight loss and carries many more health benefits.

How about you? Are you still living in a politically correct fantasy where beans, seeds, fruits and greens contain protein? Are you relying heavily on non-animal foods to provide you with a sustainable or low fat weight loss ,but instead seeing the opposite results? Do you get gas and bloating after your low protein meals? Do you see bean skins and vegetables in your stools? Are you starting to develop allergies and intolerances to other foods? If any of these apply, then I suggest you seriously consider eliminating beans and reducing copious amounts of fruit and raw vegetables from your diet and to increase your intake of animal foods from a variety of sources.

Some will undoubtedly be relieved to learn that meat is back on the menu, while others will still be intimidated or even angered by this idea. To the latter, I suggest learning to relax and to succumb to the carnal pleasures of animal foods. The drive to eat real protein is hard coded in humans no matter what we may be able to convince ourselves of.

Those who have actively avoided animal foods for a long time often experience digestive problems upon reintroduction. This is due to an evolutionary mechanism that shuts down digestive juice production in the absence of protein. To get back on track, I suggest visiting the Nutrition Heretic website at http://nutritionheretic.com for one of my upcoming digestion repair workshops.

Tip #2: Slippery When Wet

To French your food properly, you want the experience to be pleasantly moist, not sopping wet. Few things are a bigger turn off than being slobbered on during a romantic encounter.

I first learned about the dangers of drinking too much water from Madame Claudine. The danger of drinking too much water is one of two very valuable tips she gave me during my stay that has stuck with me all these years.

As the story goes, we were sitting around the lunch table on this particular day when my doughy, pimple-faced roommate and I (whose skin was only marginally better at the time) turned the conversation toward the virtues of drinking lots of water. We were bragging about drinking a liter (roughly a quart) or more per day (conservative by today's standards), when the old lady dropped this bomb on us. "Be careful with water!", she said, "If you drink too much, your body will go into shock and you could die!"

My roommate and I looked at her as if she was ready for the old folks home. Who the heck was she kidding? Everybody knows that you can't overdo water! Silly, old-fashioned French lady! What the heck does *she* know?

As it turns out, she knew a lot more than we gave her credit for. Years later with a few nutrition degrees under my belt, I realize that she was 100% right and we were miserably wrong. While drinking water is certainly better than drinking soda, juice, alcohol or coffee, it does not mean that there are no limits. It is a tragedy that most Americans have embraced the standard eight-by-eight recommendation (to drink eight ounces of water eight times per day) without questioning the practice. I even received hate mail from followers of what I call the "Cult of Unlimited Water Consumption", when I first wrote publicly about this topic in my book, *Drowning in 8 Glasses*.

Even more disturbing is that many people have independently decided that this recommendation is on the low side, aiming to fit as much water into their bodies as possible. This advice has landed many people in a coma and caused several deaths.

There are many reasons why this advice systematically fails many people. One is because the water we drink is devoid of minerals. Another is because we guzzle our water because otherwise it is hard to fit that much in. And third, it puts our kidneys under a lot of strain to work continuously to pump all of that water.

Our kidneys are responsible for removing certain toxins out of our body and do use water and minerals for this function, but it is ridiculous to assume that they do not need a period of relative rest for performing other functions. The adrenal glands, which sit atop the kidneys use hormone secretions to tell the kidneys what to do and when to do it—such as maintaining mineral balance by exchanging sodium and potassium as well as managing stress. Therefore, flooding the kidneys with water not only depletes minerals, potentially sending the body into shock, but also adds stress to these already busy organs, often resulting in premature graying (as a former water guzzler, I can attest to this!).

Indeed, it is highly unusual to see French women carrying water bottles with them everywhere they go. Even in office settings, I have not seen this practice. However in situations where they know they will be losing a lot of water -- for example, at the beach or on a hike -- they are inclined to carry water with them as opposed to the Gatorade-type drinks that Americans often opt for.

The type of water the French drink is generally different too. Here in the States, the focus is on "clean water with nothing in it". Little attention, if any, is paid to mineral content. In my opinion, mineral content is the real reason we should drink water.

In France, if you order a bottle of mineral water in a restaurant, you are asked if you want it flat or sparkling. Then you are presented with a bottle of water that proudly boasts its mineral content on the label.

On the other hand, if you order mineral water in an American restaurant, it is not uncommon to be asked to explain what mineral water is. If you describe it as sparkling water, you are more than likely presented with a bottle of seltzer or club soda, which are not only devoid of minerals, but taste awful. That is not to say that American restaurants do not carry mineral water. Many do. Those places sadly are not the norm. American restaurants have a lot to catch up with in this regard.

So if you want to drink water like the French do, consider adding sparkling mineral water to your diet. Each brand tastes different, so try a few before deciding whether or not you like it. Over the years, many clients, friends and family members have successfully and easily given up sodas simply by switching to sparkling mineral water. When your body gets the nutrition it needs, ditching processed junk is easy! As a bonus, many women who suffer from PMS-related cramping and fatigue may find that drinking mineral water stops the cramps and fatigue in their tracks.

Other than mineral water, another way that the French get adequate water into their diet is from the foods they eat. Vegetables, meats, milk and fruits are 65 to 90% water, while grains—a relatively small part of their diet—provide less than 50%. Freshly made soups, especially those made from real soup stock, are a potent source of both water and minerals. The French often have a bowl of soup with or as a meal, particularly in the evening. Snack foods like potato chips, crackers, cookies and pretzels, on the other hand, contain virtually no water -- one of many very good reasons to avoid them.

It is not uncommon for a French person to have yogurt with an egg and a piece of fruit for breakfast, a salad with fish or a soup for lunch and a rare steak with vegetables for dinner with perhaps a piece of fruit for dessert. These are all prime sources of water in perfect balance with the minerals contained in food. To round out their water requirement, they sip small amounts of water or herbal teas whenever they need a break. They do like a shot of espresso once or twice per day in a café or sometimes a bowl (not cup) of coffee at home, but that's usually all as far as it goes for caffeinated beverages.

Suzanna, a new mother, is the perfect example of

someone who nearly killed herself with excess water consumption. Shortly after giving birth, Suzanna developed a urinary tract infection and was urged by a local nurse practitioner to drink more water as part of her treatment. The nurse practitioner, unfortunately, did not take into account that Suzanna was on a low-fat, vegan diet -- a diet that is naturally high in carbohydrates (a primary cause of urinary tract infections) and low in sodium. So within three days of increasing her water intake to eight glasses or more per day, Suzanna slipped into a coma. Fortunately, over the week that followed, doctors were able to bring her sodium levels back to within normal range and she eventually recovered. If you have also been convinced that eight glasses of water or more cannot be dangerous, then I urge you to consider Suzanna's case plus the wisdom of the French and listen to your body instead of blanket recommendations disseminated by bottled water companies.

Another consideration with water is that it is best to drink away from meals. Why? Because drinking water during meals dilutes digestive juices. This leads to inadequate digestion of food and eventually turns into food allergies and intolerances.

To summarize, tip number two is to drink water with grace and dignity. Don't fall prone to becoming a water slut. Learn to French with just enough moisture.

You can learn more about the dangers of too much water as well as how to properly ingest water in _Drowning in 8 Glasses_ on Amazon.com.

Tip #3: Porking It

How crude I found her when Madame Claudine tried to coerce us into taking part is such a disgusting and vulgar practice. Not only did she find drinking less water a turn on, now she was trying to convince us of the unthinkable -- that lard is better for us than butter and even olive oil!

My (non-practicing) Jewish roommate was particularly horrified by this concept. Neither he nor I were the picture of health, yet we immediately went into defense mode promoting the benefits of vegetable oils (not just olive) over any animal fats, but especially *lard*. Didn't this 70-year old woman who had been eating lard all her life know that it could kill her? It sounds ridiculous to think of it this way now, but at the time, I was really convinced that she had somehow defied nature instead of recognizing that her longevity was a testament to the benefits of lard.

What she replied, however, has stuck with me now for all these years. She said "Pork fat is much *lighter* than butter. It is easier for the body to digest." Compared to olive oil, she told us that "Olive oil causes wrinkles and can make you fat. Lard doesn't."

Making digestion easy for the body is a concept that few people in the United States consider. Our assessment of how our bodies interact with food falls into two categories: good and bad. Little attention is paid to quality, pacing or physiological need.

Today when I think of her sage advice, my mind immediately goes to the light and sensual nature of a perfectly baked lard pie crust. It is one of the most pleasurable eating experiences on the planet that few Americans today have had the pleasure of enjoying. It is not only lighter in texture, but does not sit like a rock in your belly because, unless you have a pork allergy or other digestive damage, is easy to digest.

Yet the mere mention of the word 'lard', and the average American starts imagining visions of arteries spontaneously clogging. Don't think for a minute that the vegetable oil industry (the guys who bring us canola, soy, corn and other industrialized fake oils) doesn't want it that way! They invented this image! And they continue to make billions of dollars off of this convenient lie. The sale of these rancid vegetable oils, diet programs, non-stick pans, microwaves, many medical procedures and drugs to treat almost everything from infertility to heart disease and more have benefited from vilifying lard and other animal fats.

It is not uncommon for people who switch exclusively to olive oil or other vegetable oils to get frustrated with their waistlines or see the signs of aging take over practically overnight. Yet they never consider that olive oil could be the cause because they have heard nothing, but the supposed benefits of consuming it.

It is sad that many people have already made up their minds (as I once had) that animal fats are bad. The few that eventually begin to understand the dangers of vegetable oils, end up typically opt to avoid all fats and oils instead of switching to or incorporating animal fats into the diet.

Unbeknownst to them, animal fats have many benefits such as regulating metabolism, improving vitamin and mineral uptake and even preventing constipation. Plus, when it comes from pigs raised on pasture instead of grain, lard is one of nature's most potent sources of vitamin D.

The French are not the only ones who revere pig fat for its many virtues. The Italians prize *lardo*, a kind of fatback seasoned with herbs and spices, so much that there is still an annual festival celebrating it. The Chinese recognize it for its health promoting properties including its use in curing constipation. Even the Okinawans, whom we are often told eat mainly soybeans and rice with small amounts of fish, routinely cook their food in lard -- a fact I first learned from several Japanese friends including one who had trouble locating fresh, non-hydrogenated lard during the years she lived in the U.S.

Keep in mind that Madame Claudine did not say that butter or olive oil were bad for the body. She merely pointed out that lard was easier to digest. So consider not taking the typical American approach of complete avoidance by dumping all other fats and oils in favor of lard. Rather, try to eat a combination of real fats and oils, each of which carries its own health benefits.

Frenching with lard and other animal fats is sexy. It keeps you slim, looking young and living long.

Tip #4: Pass the Lube

When your Frenching gets to a heated state of passion, it is only logical that you start to get a little moist. You don't want it to end. You want it to go on until you're completely satisfied.

So often, Americans cut our satisfaction short at mealtime. Afraid of falling into sin, we choose a less-than-satisfactory route for our carnal pleasures. The result is often overeating of synthetic, addictive and sickeningly sweet replacements for the real foods that our bodies desire.

As I said previously, when I was learning to French at the newspaper, not a week went by where we weren't swapping diet techniques. Eventually many of the men got sucked into the frenzy as well. My French colleagues living in New York were just beginning to start fearing fat much like the average American.

One little tip they shared though, left me baffled for years afterward -- even after I began embracing fat for all its virtues. They insisted that mustard was fattening, but that mayonnaise wasn't!

The French have a great tradition of eating both mayonnaise and mustard, so how (I wondered) could they miss the obvious -- that fat makes you fat and anything without fat doesn't?

Then one day—not that long ago actually—it dawned on me. Mustard contains goitrogens! Goitrogens block iodine uptake to the thyroid. The thyroid regulates metabolism and iodine is crucial to its proper function. Without adequate iodine feeding the thyroid, thyroid function is impaired and we get fat. This is why many practitioners dabbling in nutrition often prescribe iodine as a first line remedy to people with hypothyroidism (however this rarely works on its own since there are many reasons for and types of hypothyroidism as there are additional nutrients that are important to the thyroid gland's use of iodine).

There are many foods that are goitrogenic: anything in the mustard family also known as crucifers including kale, cabbage, broccoli, brussel sprouts and cauliflower; soybeans; peas; peanuts; radishes; and spinach. These foods should be eaten only in relatively small amounts and ALWAYS cooked or fermented. Cooking and fermenting not only significantly reduce the goitrogenic activity of these foods, but they make them much easier to digest and liberate the nutrients bound inside the cell walls too. In the case of soybeans, cooking is not enough to remove the goitrogens and they must be fermented to make them safe enough not to inhibit thyroid function. Even so, the amount of fermented soy products is best left at a tablespoon or less per day.

When I was diagnosed with hypothyroidism about 20 years ago, the first thing I learned was to eliminate these goitrogenic foods, while my thyroid healed. Today, hypothyroidism affects more than 11 million Americans and that number is rising, yet many of our health trends—such as the amount of soy lurking in almost every food product on the market as well as the push to eat kale as the new beef for its iron content—do not consider the repercussions of eating such an unbalanced diet. Given this information about goitrogens, would you still think it is so wise to avoid animal foods in favor of such substitutes?

Although mayonnaise does contain a small amount of mustard, its combination with good quality eggs, olive oil, and vinegar help the body to uptake many minerals and vitamins while lubricating and nourishing the mucous membranes. Be aware that most mayonnaise in North America that is made from canola or soybean oil. We have already looked at the goitrogenic nature of soy, but canola—even in its organic form—is genetically altered. Unless you enjoy being the guinea pig for corporations to make money from you at the expense of your health, it is worth it to pay a few dollars extra for one made with olive oil. If you can get one that uses red wine vinegar instead of distilled grain vinegar, even better still. Distilled vinegar, canola and soybean oil do not have the health promoting properties of the real mayo that the French enjoy.

Real mayonnaise is the perfect moistening agent to an otherwise dry sandwich. It also provides necessary cholesterol from the egg yolks to nourish your brain and spinal chord. Above all, it satisfies so that you are less likely to run searching for a piece of cake later. It is good stuff, so it is totally worth it to seek it out or make your own!!

Whatever you do, please don't take this advice as a manifesto against mustard. Mustard is delicious and a great compliment to very many foods. However, if you're struggling with your weight, you may want to consider mayo instead.

Tip #5: The Raw Beef Injection

My friend, Brigitte, who lives on the tiny Caribbean island of St. Martin, can French like no one I've ever met before. At 50 years old, she has a body and face that any woman of any age would kill for.

During one of our routine conversations about food, I told her how worried I was about a friend who had recently embraced a raw food diet even though she was not thriving on it. Brigitte gasped and put her hand to her mouth. Then she blurted out, "But that causes all kinds of gas! You can't digest that!"

It's true. Many advocates of raw diets, especially those that exclude all animal foods, suffer from abdominal distention and are able to recognize foods in their stools. A quick Google search of phrases such as "food in stools" reveals approximately 17 million results, many of which come from raw food enthusiasts asking questions about what they see in the toilet and their other digestive woes. French women like Brigitte know that food should be fully digested and that an upset stomach and bloating after a meal are not normal.

Just as cruciferous vegetables need cooking, so do many foods in the human diet. Humans are not like other animals. We need many foods to be cooked in order to make the nutrients in the cells usable by the body. This applies particularly to vegetables and starches. Many historians and health researchers have concluded that the advent of cooking both animal and vegetable foods marked a huge leap in human brain development. The French, thankfully, still largely understand this.

Ironically, the foods that we normally think of as always needing to be cooked, meat and dairy, can actually be better for you when consumed raw. In fact, the French still understand this too with steak tartare, tuna carpaccio and raw milk cheeses appearing frequently on menus and on supermarket shelves. On a personal note, I have found that eating raw fish and beef improves my digestion of grain-based foods like bread and rice – so carbs are back on the menu!

The French often eat a portion of their animal foods raw, while eating a small amount of salad and perhaps a piece of fruit as their raw serving for the day. Other than that, much of their diet is carefully cooked.

With so many people embracing the local food movement, I am surprised at how many people have jumped on the raw food bandwagon -- especially those living in cold climates. Eating a diet comprised of all or even mostly raw foods not only overlooks the fact that much of the nutrition remains bound in the cell walls of the vegetables, but it also overlooks the fact that our bodies are ever-changing because of the aging process as well as external conditions such as climate.

Most every culture understands this, but the Chinese understand this so perfectly that it is a rule in Chinese medicine: when it is cold outside, eat more cooked and warming foods. Eating all raw foods all the time, especially when you live in a region with varying extreme climates, leads to a multitude of imbalances as the body has to work harder during colder months to maintain homeostasis.

Yet even in consistently warm climates, people still cook their food. The Chinese also see this as a way of maintaining homeostasis by causing the body to sweat, releasing toxins and cooling the body.

During the warm summer months, the French often eat a combination of raw and cooked vegetables along with grilled, rare or raw meats. In winter, they enjoy warming soups, stews and roasts with starchier accompaniments such as potatoes, beans and winter squashes.

If you have been forcing yourself to eat more raw vegetables because of some belief that it is the way food was intended to be eaten, rest assured that your urge to eat cooked vegetables is normal, natural and even necessary -- particularly where climate changes and nutrient uptake are concerned. It is okay to listen to your body even when it conflicts with what the experts say.

If you already enjoy sushi, then you've got this Frenching technique under your belt. However, if you've been trained to fear potential parasitic infection from raw meat, you may need to ease into this practice. Freezing your meat for two weeks prior to consumption is said to kill any pathogens and may be an option worth exploring. All I can say is that I have been Frenching with raw meat and dairy for more than 15 years and not once have I had even a remotely bad experience.

Tip #6: Slow and Comfortable

When most people conjure up images of a French woman, chances are she is not killing herself on a treadmill or doing *The Insanity Workout*. More than likely, she is lounging on the beach or sitting in a café without a care in the world.

This is not to imply that French women do not move. It is not uncommon to see French women taking a leisurely stroll through the streets of Paris, running around to do their shopping or taking a leisurely bike ride down a country lane. In a 2012 interview with travel host Rick Steves, French author, Olivier Magny, summed it up best; "A good majority of people who jog in Paris are foreigners. The French don't really exercise much. They basically look down on people who do to be perfectly honest. The only exception you'll find is Parisians who have spent time in the U.S."

Instead of spending hours running or at the gym, they would much rather spend time preparing and sitting down to a great meal. The French spend hours every day talking about and planning their menus. This is one thing that Mireille Guiliano and I agree on. When the time to eat comes, they like to sit down with their friends and families and spend at least an hour enjoying one another's company. Frenching your food is a relaxing experience. For the most part it is not filled with anxiety and fear as it is in the States.

In America, we often treat meals as if they are part of some race to get the dirty, shameful deed done and over with as fast as possible. By not planning our meals or thinking about where they will come from, we often end up making poor, last minute choices in the form of take out, frozen meals or even snacking on chips, pretzels or some other non-nutritive form of empty calories.

Sometimes we do not even want to stop what we are doing to eat. Some people read a book, work on the computer or watch TV routinely during meals (I am often guilty of the last one). Some take it a step further and end up eating while standing over the sink instead of grabbing a plate and sitting down to eat in a relaxed setting. It is almost as if we think that by not focusing on our meals and enjoying them we are tricking our bodies into thinking that we are not consuming this evil source of calories. Can you imagine where our human relationships would be, if we treated them all with the same disdain with which we treat our food?

As our collective food shame drives us to consume more processed replacement "foods", our nation's health and weight are spiraling out of control. Health authorities are at their wits' end to find a way to at least curb the resultant weight issue. For this reason, they have turned to exercise as a failsafe for this problem.

Where they miss the mark, in my opinion, is by misleading us into thinking that exercise will solve not only the weight issue, but also all other health issues by somehow infusing our bodies with nutrients that are not present in the diet. For this reason, I have seen many lay people and health practitioners alike prioritize exercise over all other components of a healthy lifestyle. In this way, it is not very different from the eight-by-eight water recommendations.

Many people seem to think that they can beat their bodies into submission and force themselves to lose weight by doing hours upon hours of exercise every day at the expense of balanced meals and even sleep! While some people will appear to correct conditions like diabetes with this regimen in the short term, there is frequently a rebound effect, which leaves them frustrated and confused. As a result, they become obsessed with working out even more often to the complete exclusion of all other health promoting activities.

Recently a very overweight aerobics teacher client of mine, who teaches 14 hours of high-intensity classes per week excluding her mentoring and other classes, decided to consult an Ayurvedic practitioner because she found my regimen of eating real food and curbing her teaching schedule a bit too "off-the-wall". This practitioner, a Westerner trained in an Americanized version of Ayurveda, told her that her weight problems were primarily due to inactivity and laziness! This woman's work schedule is already so busy that she barely has enough time to grab a slice of pizza before teaching. Additionally, she suffers from joint pain and is unable to sleep at night even though she was completely fatigued from her schedule. Surely, most people of average weight or even skinny people do not work out for 14 hours or more per week. I know I don't. So is it wise to assume that even *more* exercise would work?

What most people, self-educated health practitioners and even medical doctors do not realize is that continuous strenuous exercise can easily become a stressor over time.

Combine that with stress from work, poor diet, lack of sleep, raising children, paying bills and all the other stresses that people deal with, and excessive exercise is more likely to do harm than good.

Remember in the section about drinking water where we discussed the role of the adrenal glands in stress management? The adrenals kick into action in times of acute stress. As cave dwellers, they would have shunted our energy normally used for digestion, maintaining a steady heart beat, and keeping our nerves calm to our brains and limbs so that we could think quick on our feet while sprinting away from a ferocious prehistoric animal.

Today, however, it seems that we never stop running from wild animals because the stress is prolonged, even ingrained in our lifestyle as it comes at us from so many different directions simultaneously. This leads to the adrenals working overtime to save us from death instead of allowing our bodies to digest our food and help us to feel safe. Do we really need to add more fuel to the fire by exercising indiscriminately?

Only a handful of health practitioners seem to recognize the fact that the adrenals also work in tandem with the thyroid. If you remember from earlier, the thyroid controls our metabolism. Here's how it works. When the adrenals are under continuous stress (from too much water, exercise or other "wild animals"), the thyroid goes into overdrive to provide the energy normally handled by the adrenals. When the thyroid has been taxed by things like the excess intake of goitrogens, the adrenals step in to help with the thyroid crisis. So what, then, should we expect to happen when both the adrenals and the thyroid are being continuously challenged by too much water, an overload of soybeans, and constantly running as if to save our lives?

In recognizing the reciprocal relationship of these glands, it becomes crystal clear that relaxation may in fact be one way to boost the metabolism by allowing each organ to perform its primary function unencumbered. If we learn to respect their needs while nourishing them, they will be able to function as close to full capacity as possible.

To exercise enthusiasts, this will seem like heresy, but don't jump to conclusions. My intent is not to vilify exercise. It is to draw attention to the fact that it is actually possible to overdo exercise when performed for extended periods of time. The new trends in exercise, such as the 15-minute per week workout described in Timothy Ferriss's book, *The Four-Hour Body*, underscore the benefits of long periods of relaxation in between bursts of exercise.

The fact remains that the average French woman does not exhaust herself with high-intensity exercise yet maintains a slim figure and is more likely to make it to 100 years of age than the average American woman. So if crazy and exhausting workouts are not yielding the results you are looking for, then consider doing the opposite by taking a cue from the French, even if just for a few weeks to observe the results.

First, reduce or even cut out exercise and opt for more leisurely activities to move your body. Take a refreshing bike ride on a secluded path, walk and window shop with a friend, clean your house or spend the day cooking a lovely meal.

Next, spend time really thinking about your meals. Give

some forethought to delicious food that makes your mouth water no matter how sinful your peers think it is. It does not need to be fancy, just real food that is treated with respect. Use real dishes, even china if you have some (often vintage china can be found at consignment shops and the Salvation Army store for pennies per piece). Paper and plastic plates or utensils have no place at a table where you plan to honor your food lover.

At meals, turn on enjoyable, soothing music or listen to a radio show that is calming, not aggravating. If you are eating with someone else, take time to get to know each other. Discuss the events of the day, make plans for an upcoming vacation or tell jokes. The point is to leave the stresses of the day somewhere else. Don't bring them to meals. Meals are a time for invigorating sustenance, not for upsetting news.

Make sure you take time to do absolutely nothing even if just for a few minutes each day. In France, as well as in other parts of the world where people are skinny, it is common to see people sitting around the house or in cafés chatting with each other for hours at a time. This relaxation time combined with an adequate sleep regimen of at least seven hours of sleep each night are important to your body's ability to repair itself. If you cannot get seven hours at one time, then try to set aside at least half an hour during the day to close your eyes for a quick pick me up. My friend, Brigitte—the one with the killer body—and her husband swear by the health promoting properties of adequate rest and relaxation.

After a time of feeling safe from being chased by the previously mentioned prehistoric animal and eating nourishing foods, the body will naturally begin to shed excess pounds (unless there are some other issues involved such as yeast overgrowth, hypothyroidism, heavy metal toxicity or food allergies). In some cases, the damage from prolonged overexercise and poor food choices is too great for the body to overcome on its own. If this is your situation, then consider finding a practitioner trained in healing adrenal fatigue or visit the Nutrition Heretic website to keep up with adrenal fatigue healing modalities.

Tip #7: Ménage à Trois

French women routinely eat meals. As is done in many cultures around the world, they eat three of them every day and unlike Americans, don't have snacks scripted into their daily routine.

That is not to say that the French do not enjoy an occasional snack. It is just not an expected part of the day. A public service announcement currently running on the French children's television station, *Gulli*, reinforces this idea by urging children to avoid routine snacking to promote a healthy weight.

In contrast, here in the United States, it has become increasingly popular to promote the idea of snacking or grazing (eating 5 or more small meals) throughout the day over three meals per day. Originally a recommendation for diabetics and others with blood sugar management issues, now nearly all fitness and health enthusiasts recommend this snacking tactic for everyone. The rationale is that sitting down to eat "three big meals" is too taxing on the digestive system and essentially that the whole world, including French women, has it wrong.

So which works better? Three meals or all-day snacking? To answer these questions, we need to look at the reasoning behind them.

To the French, eating is about pleasure, sustenance and community. As I mentioned before, they spend hours every day thinking about, planning and eating meals. Whenever possible meals are consumed in a relaxed setting being eaten slowly and deliberately. Snacking is rare and is typically limited to a small piece of fruit, a square of dark chocolate or a wedge of raw milk cheese. The approach tends to keep blood sugar stable while allowing them to accomplish their work for the day. You may want to look at this as spurts of intense work (whether physical or mental) followed by long periods of relaxation. Sound familiar?

As previously mentioned, the idea of grazing was originally a recommendation aimed at diabetics and others who suffered from unstable blood sugar levels. Eating this way can indeed appear to keep people on an even keel by preventing mood swings and sudden exhaustion brought on by sudden spikes in blood sugar followed by rapidly dropping blood sugar levels. As it turns out, leveling out these highs and lows in blood sugar can also lead to weight loss.

With little exception, however, most proponents of the grazing method of weight loss are also endorsing an extremely low fat diet. It is based upon a simplistic theory that says "fat makes you fat". What they fail to realize or acknowledge is that fat, particularly saturated fat from animals and tropical oils, performs an important role in controlling the rate at which the body's cells process sugar. Without getting too technical, eating fat—real fat, not rancid plasticized oils like canola, soy and corn oil—is one of the most effective ways of controlling sudden blood sugar spikes and achieving easy weight loss.

Fats also keep us satisfied between meals. So even though fats contain more calories per gram (nine versus five calories in protein and carbohydrate), you are likely to consume fewer calories and lose weight by eating some fat and skipping snack time!

It is not uncommon to meet a very overweight person who is touting the benefits of eating five or more meals per day. "I just don't get why some people think you should just eat three meals per day," they say, "It's the worst thing for you. That's why everybody is so fat!" Looking at the amount of excess weight they are carrying, it would appear that the person feels that by saying it more, they are convincing others that their condition merely runs in the family or is otherwise beyond their control.

Such was the case with Wendie. Wendie was a swimming instructor, who had fully embraced the low-fat lifestyle. One day she came to me about her insatiable appetite. She complained that she had trouble shedding weight, but also that she could never fathom restricting her diet to only three meals per day because if she did not eat every 90 minutes, she would become grouchy and irritable. The eating had gotten particularly bad since her pregnancy when she was diagnosed with gestational diabetes and put on a special no fat diet (the worst thing for a pregnant woman or a diabetic).

Then she made a confession: she had eaten a whole avocado the day before. Wendie was terrified of the weight gain and heart attack she expected as a result of her wicked dietary choice. She wanted to know how she might be able to curb her appetite for eating fat and go longer between meals so that she could be productive.

Despite her activity level and the fact that she was only 35, it was true that Wendie was out of shape and dumpy. The skin on her face, arms and middle sagged as you might expect of a woman 20 years older. She had trouble staying awake during the day so much that she drank diet sodas from early in the morning until bedtime. I explained to her that she was constantly hungry because she was not getting any fat in her body and that the urge to eat an entire avocado was not her body betraying her with a fat craving, but her body screaming out for something that would end the "fat famine".

I suggested that she start increasing her fat intake with coconut oil and animal fats daily while cutting back on swimming for two weeks. Coconut is usually easy for people to digest because it bypasses the gallbladder where fats are initially digested, so she was able to dive in and eat to her heart's content. I had her introduce the animal fats more slowly because her gallbladder would have to relearn how to digest them after such a long period of avoidance. She made an appointment to come back and see me after the two week period had passed.

A week later, Wendie called me excited that as soon as she started eating fat, she was able to go more than 3 hours between meals *and* that her clothes were fitting better. Wendie went on to explore and enjoy the types of "rich" foods that the French are so well known for and never looked back. She also lost weight, stabilized her blood sugar effortlessly, got more done during the day without having to stop every 90 minutes to eat and her skin began to firm as well.

Wendie's situation is very typical. She was a fitness enthusiasts who had been self-educated by reading popular websites on the internet and following the standard dogma recommended by the ADA, trendy weight loss programs and coaches that only reveal one small part of the picture. All too many people have gone down this road only to end up disappointed one way or another.

My biggest issue with snacking, however, is the bad habit that it creates, which over time becomes almost impossible to adhere to in the modern era. Let me explain.

Many people implement the extra meals as part of a fairly nutritious diet plan that favors fruits and vegetables over Cup o' Soup® and Lunchables®. Over time, however, even if some weight is lost, the habit of eating the extra meal stays. Eventually, most people determine that carrying a piece of fruit, bag of celery or whatever the nutritious extra meal consisted is a nuisance or they look at the snack as a daily opportunity to "cheat" on their food. As a result, people often end up grabbing bags of chips, pretzels, rice cakes and other low-fat, low quality, highly processed snacks. They find themselves in the same cycle they had before of unconscious eating. When the fat starts packing on again, they begin to think that they have some "inherited problem" and give up on their health goals altogether. That is not only a shame, it is unnecessary.

In order to French like the French, consider making your encounters with food deliberate and meaningful. Eat more than three times per day and even the most passionate relationship can become a boring routine. Treat your food like you do your most important relationships and food will continue to honor you.

Tongue Wrestling

For Americans, the relationship with food has become an uncomfortable one of self-doubt, self-loathing and struggle. This is where I believe the real differences lie between the way we eat and how the French approach food. Reconciling these differences will send many to wrestle with their emotional and even egoic attachments to what they believe they already know about food.

A lifetime of being lied to by the bad boy diet with its promises of saving your life and making you thin will not be easily undone for most people. It will be darn near impossible for some not to be swayed by the highly processed, factory-made products that bear labels boasting "new", "improved", "nonfat", "high protein", "low cholesterol", "zero calorie", "sugar-free" and other bogus claims that bombard our lives and airwaves. If you're reading this book, however, then you are still searching for a diet that will tell you the truth. Personally, I think that Frenching, as outlined in this book, is the perfect place to start.

To summarize what you have already read, Frenching does not include a low-fat, super-restrictive lifestyle that revolves around self-deprivation and shame as has become so popular in the States. The French bring passion and excitement to their meals. In many ways, food is another person in their lives – a person who brings them joy, comfort and peace of mind, not one who brings anxiety, shame and guilt.

Even worse, the diet that scares us away from real foods such as meat, dairy, grains, fats, salt, and occasionally certain legumes, vegetables and cane sugar, sends us running toward fake garbage that is really not fit for human or animal consumption. This has not only betrayed a great number of weight loss seekers, it has resulted in a host of eating disorders and increases in diseases such as diabetes, cancer, arthritis, food allergies and has even created many new diseases. Why would we consciously choose an abusive relationship, when we can opt for a loving one that fulfills us in every way?

If you have been reading the rest of the book closely (and I believe you have been), you will have noticed that French women eat foods that take a shorter trip from the farm to table and, for the most part, have little judgments imposed on those foods. Contrary to what you may believe, they rarely spend endless hours in the kitchen, and in today's world, they do not avoid all processed foods completely. The French, however, are proud of their traditions and continue to eat many meals passed down through the generations.

Instead of seeing food as a nasty habit that must be avoided, it is more likely to be viewed as a pleasurable experience that should not be abused. True, many French women cut their portion sizes down to lose weight, but, with the exception of Mireille Guiliano's weekend leek soup diet, most of the ones that I know do not cut them as excessively as American women do. The relationship is more synergistic and less combative.

Just like any other relationship, the relationship you develop with food will be stronger and healthier once your attitude toward it changes. If you treat it as an enemy and a nuisance, everything you eat will betray you. You will make choices out of fear, not faith. Food will quickly become an ally in your health and weight loss journey, once you begin to treat it and yourself with respect. Luckily, there are only three actions you need to take to improve this relationship.

First, eating a meal is not a race. Reserve a *minimum* of 20 minutes to eat each of your meals. Do not finish in 12 and surf the net for the rest of the time. Chew each bite carefully and deliberately. Sit down, savor it and enjoy. Make it a daily treat to yourself. Try chewing each mouthful 20 to 30 times before swallowing. Your teeth are in your mouth, not in your stomach.

Next, let's take a look at our shopping list. Skinny French women are likely to shop at least every two to three days per week with Sundays off. It is part of the routine and the ritual of daily social activities and does not need to take hours to complete. A stop at the butcher on the way home from work could result in some ground beef for dinner as easily as it could mean a roast chicken. Perhaps a stop at the cheese shop or the deli means some ham, salami, some plain yogurt and a small cheese assortment (real cheese, not American cheese, which is processed). Lastly, a stop at the green grocer would be some salad items, cooking vegetables for a nice soup or mixed vegetable sauté and some fruits for dessert.

I know that here in the States, it is not easy to find a quaint little town with all of these specialty shops, but all of these items are all easily located in regular American supermarkets (or in Italian or Asian markets in slightly more diverse neighborhoods), so there is no excuse not to start today. One caveat is that American versions of things like yogurt may contain additives that would not be in the French equivalent. So if possible, get one made only with whole milk and cultures. If you cannot find one without additives or that is made from skim milk, don't sweat it. Better to eat a decent quality yogurt than a muffin or granola bar that contains all calories and zero nutrition.

So let's see what a sample menu might look like:

Breakfast

One egg: soft-boiled, fried over easy or scrambled soft

A six ounce serving of plain yogurt with fresh berries and a little honey added

A small piece of baguette with butter and jam (optional)

A shot of espresso or bowl of coffee (typically without milk)

Lunch

One *salade niçoise:* green salad with olives, canned tuna, tomatoes, cucumbers and hard boiled eggs

Glass of sparkling mineral water

An orange, kiwi or other small piece of fruit for dessert

Dinner

One pan-fried lamb chop or a few slices of roast lamb

Mushrooms sautéed with garlic, olive oil and chopped parsley

Small roasted potato

Glass of sparkling mineral water or mint tea

Fruit salad

Here's another one:

Breakfast

A few pieces of baguette with pâté

Slices of tomato

Shot of espresso or bowl of coffee

Lunch (in a restaurant)

Carpaccio (raw beef slices) or a small steak (approx. 4-6 ounces) cooked rare with small portion of fries

Small green salad

Shot of espresso, a small coffee and/or mineral water

Snack

Two to three small squares of chocolate or a piece of cheese

Dinner

Bowl of tomato soup with Swiss cheese shreds and a few croutons

A small fruit tart or yogurt

Glass of sparkling mineral water or mint tea

As you can see, lunch is often the biggest meal of the day -- although this is shifting with rigid work hours preventing people from enjoying their midday breaks. These meals are also not complicated and if you get organized, they can take less time to get on the table and clean up after than ordering from the place down the corner that delivers. Let the whole family join in, while you create great memories to last a lifetime.

I am always reminded of how simple skinny French women make it their business to eat well whenever I attend a potluck dinner and monthly get togethers at the local French club. At French affairs, the food is rich and inviting: *pâtés*; sliced ham or salami; stuffed hardboiled eggs; well-dressed green salads with olives, anchovies and tomatoes; tender and juicy chicken dishes; *foie gras*; finger sandwiches; quiches; cheese platters; fruit platters; beautiful fruit tarts; and chocolate mousse. Each item on the table is a taste sensation that puts a smile on my face and gets my juices flowing.

At American gatherings, the experience is quite different. Textured vegetable protein, tater tots, fake cheeses (including American cheese, as well as soy and almond-based cheese alternatives), multiple renditions of grain and other starch-based such as pasta, quinoa and rice salads as well as bean dishes and relatively few vegetables and salads, which is a bit of a let down when you live in a community of people who consider themselves health-conscious.

Well-meaning individuals go the extra mile to make sure that nearly every ounce of fat and salt has been removed, leaving many of the dishes lacking in sustenance and flavor. Often more than half the table is weighed down with dessert items at American gatherings. Cakes, muffins and cookies make up the bulk of the desserts, while an occasional fruit pie and some watermelon slices round out the selection. Sadly, despite all the effort to do "the right thing", a large number of these people suffer from overweight, advanced aging and even more serious conditions such as diabetes and cancer. All of which could most likely be avoided by a more nutritious diet. Indeed, I have seen far less of these disorders (almost zero, in fact) in the French communities I frequent.

Keep in mind that the above is a generalization. On occasion, someone who does not have time to cook may stop by the supermarket to pick up a cheese or fruit platter on the way. And even more infrequently, there is someone who may bring a crockpot with something flavorful like fried rice or a nicely flavored (i.e. adequately salted) stew or a meat dish. Unfortunately, these are the exception, not the norm.

You don't need to be a great chef to prepare the kinds of foods that are appropriate for Frenching. You don't even need to like cooking. Many French women don't (even though they love to talk about food). My point here is to illustrate (yet again) that while we are killing ourselves to do the right thing, we are ignoring the fact that skinny French women achieve their great figures and good health almost effortlessly while enjoying real, nourishing and satisfying food.

The third action is to love yourself. Many times throughout this book, I have made references to the bad boy diet shaming us into self-hatred and lowered self-esteem. If you want to change this dynamic and develop a healthy relationship with your body and your food, then know deep in your heart that you are *worth it!* You deserve to nourish your body with the best foods that your pocket book can afford. You deserve the best health. You deserve to love yourself, even if you have some dimples, wrinkles, a flat chest and thunder thighs. You deserve to put yourself on a pedestal every time you open your mouth to eat.

Before I met my husband, I went through a string of less-than-fulfilling relationships from a guy who pined for his ex-girlfriend to another guy who wanted to marry me for a visa to stay in the United States. I put up with it because these were the types of relationships I saw around me and so to me, they seemed relatively normal.

One day, however, I got sick of it. I met someone who made me realize that there were better people out in the world for me. This realization empowered me to begin caring for myself. I bought myself nice clothes, took dance classes for fun, went shopping for incense and candles, meditated, took long hot bubble baths on the weekends and focused on treating myself like a queen. Within one month, I met my husband, who instinctively treated me like I was the sexiest woman he had ever met. We have been together now for almost 20 years.

Since then, I have taught many women in difficult relationships to learn how to honor themselves and the results have been staggering. Some deadbeat husbands clean up their acts and begin to respect and treat them better, while other cheating boyfriends get out of the way to let a new, more satisfying relationship take its place.

It is no different with food. Giving up the cycle of falling for every starvation fad in favor of Frenching has the capacity to improve your mood, give you more confidence in any situation, boost your immunity and put *more money* in your pocket. That's right! Every person I have taught to French has ended up telling me that they were richer after learning to French.

This happens for two reasons. The first reason is because they don't get sick so often and have more mental clarity, they make more money in their jobs and get more promotions. Second is that they aren't buying all of the expensive diet crap and snack garbage any longer, so even if they spend more per meal, they aren't throwing money away by buying into all the diet fads around them.

Don't take this advice lightly. This works! Start Frenching and you will set the foundation to embrace a fulfilling relationship that you can carry forward for the rest of your life.

Getting It from Both Ends

In more recent years, it has been sad to note that even many skinny French women have become swayed by American ideas of weight loss and health. For example, even though the French have enjoyed a robust dairy tradition throughout centuries which has worked well for them, French health food stores are now beginning to push dairy replacements especially rice and soy milk. I find this trend rather curious as the French have never really consumed milk as a beverage even though they have eaten (and largely continue to eat) butter, cheese and yogurt. They know that they live longer than us and are slimmer, so why are they looking for milk replacements? Even once completely foreign concepts, such as low-fat, vegetarian and vegan are becoming all the rage in many French people under the age of 50.

Another trend I find relatively disturbing in more recent years is the Dukan Diet, founded by Dr. Pierre Dukan. Similar to the Atkins Diet, the Dukan Diet promises rapid weight loss. But at what cost? Where the Atkins Diet supported the consumption of important saturated fats such as butter and lard along with liberal amounts of meat (all typical elements of Frenching), the Dukan Diet is an ultra low-fat diet that while it still supports some animal protein, also endorses less nourishing options such as seitan and tofu. Only time will tell what the true outcome of a generation of women following this type of diet will bring, but I certainly would not want to be the guinea pig for such a diet.

One area where we do agree is with regards to exercise. One 30-minute brisk (or slow) walk daily is way preferable to the torturous workout schedules that are all the rage these days in our country.

Overall, however, it does appear that Dr. Dukan's approach to dieting is the typical knee-jerk reaction that many American über-low fat diets take. It appears to prioritize weight loss over crucial elements of robust health such as proper digestion and elimination which in turn control virtually all other disorders from mental health to muscular integrity.

Along with each health fad to hit the market, come all the health repercussions that are so prevalent in the United States such as depression, migraines, schizophrenia, advanced aging (i.e. wrinkling and sagging skin, early menopause etc), anxiety attacks, hypoglycemia, diabetes, and cancer. It remains to be seen how far these trends will continue before these skinny French women realize that they were doing not only fine, but better without them.

On a more personal note, I hope that this book has helped you to gain some perspective on Frenching and how it is gradually changing thanks to outside influences. I wish you the best of luck on your journey. If you feel you have learned something helpful in this book, then please leave a review at Amazon.com. Also, I would love to offer you some free recipes from my newest book, *Honeylingus: 50 Healthy Honey Recipes that Will Leave You Begging for More* as well as a sneak peek at my upcoming projects, health tips to break free of worthless nutrition fads and more. Go to http://honeyling.us today to get started.

Resources

Brownstein, David, *Salt Your Way to Health*, Medical Alternative Press, 2006.

Bukisa.com, *Drinking Excess Water Can Result IN Coma And Seizures*, http://www.bukisa.com/articles/312222_drinking-excess-water-can-result-in-coma-and-seizures, 2010.

Byrnes, Stephen, *Diet & Heart Disease: It's NOT What You Think…*, Whitman Publications, 2001.

Enig, Mary, *Know Your Fats: The Complete Primer for Understanding the Nutrition of Fats, Oils, and Cholesterol*, Bethesda Press, 2000.

Ferriss, Timothy, *The 4-Hour Body: An Uncommon Guide to Rapid Fat-Loss, Incredible Sex, and Becoming Superhuman*, Harmony Books, 2010.

Fleming, D.W., S.L. Cochi, et al., *Pasteurized Milk as a Vehicle of Infection in an Outbreak of Listeriosis*, The New England Journal of Medicine, Volume 312:404-407, February 14, 1985.

Guiliano, Mireille, *French Women Don't Get Fat*, Vintage, 2007.

Guiliano, Mireille, *French Women Don't Get Fat Cookbook*, Atria, 2011.

Lu, Henry C., *Chinese Natural Cures: Traditional Methods for Remedies and Preventions*, Black Dog & Leventhal Publishers, Inc., 1994.

Monastyrsky, Konstantin, *Fiber Menace: The Truth About the Leading Role of Fiber in Diet Failure, Constipation, Hemorrhoids, Irritable Bowel Syndrome, Ulcerative Colitis, Crohn's Disease, and Colon Cancer*, Ageless Press, 2005.

Negus, George, George Negus Tonight, *Episode 18, Water Intoxication*, http://www.abc.net.au/dimensions/ dimensions_health/Transcripts/s871112.htm

Pizzorno, Joseph E. and Michael T. Murray, *Textbook of Natural Medicine*, *Churchill Livingstone*, 2000.

Wilson, James, *Adrenal Fatigue: The 21st Century Stress Syndrome*, Smart Publications, 2001.

Recommended Reading

French Women Don't Get Fat by Mireille Guiliano

French Women Don't Get Fat Cookbook by Mireille Guiliano

Know Your Fats: The Complete Primer for Understanding the Nutrition of Fats, Oils, and Cholesterol by Dr. Mary Enig

Nourishing Traditions by Sally Fallon Morell and Dr. Mary Enig
  The 4-Hour Body: An Uncommon Guide to Rapid Fat-Loss, Incredible Sex, and Becoming Superhuman by Timothy Ferriss

Books in the Health AlternaTips Series

Available at adriennehew.com

Drowning in 8 Glasses: 7 Myths about Water Revealed

Frenching Your Food: 7 Guilt-Free French Diet Tips to Slim Down, Look Younger and Live Longer without Calorie Counting or Strenuous Exercise

Books in the Affordable Organics & GMO-Free Series

Available at adriennehew.com

50 Ways to Eat Cock: Healthy Chicken Recipes with Balls!

Honeylingus: 50 Healthy Honey Recipes that Will Leave You Begging for More

Good Times, Great Food: Fighting Childhood Obesity and Picky Eating One Celebration at a Time (coming soon)

FREE GIFT

SPECIAL GIFTS FOR YOU!

Want a sneak peek at some outrageously delicious recipes that work great with *Frenching Your Food*? Looking for more information on what's safe and healthy to eat? Want *real* answers to your health questions?

Grab these recipes from my new book, *Honeylingus: 50 Healthy Honey Recipes that Will Leave You Begging for More* and more by going to http:// honeyling.us to claim your FREE gifts today!

About the Author

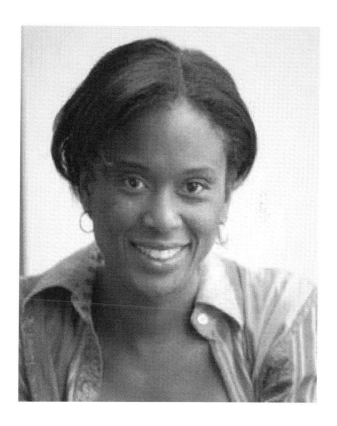

Adrienne Hew has been called "the Nutrition Heretic" and "the Pope of Health" because of the unique sense of levelheadedness she brings to discussions on nutrition. Both Dietetic Associations and politically correct, conventionally trained alternative health advocates often have difficulty reconciling their beliefs with the truth contained in her observations and experiences.

Ms. Hew began her holistic health journey after suffering innumerable health problems and near death experiences while following the American Dietetics Association's dietary recommendations. Born into a multicultural family that had thrived on a very different diet, she set on a quest to learn the dietary commonalities amongst all healthy societies. Her fluency in three languages has enabled her to uncover many long forgotten food traditions throughout the world.

Receiving a certificate in Chinese dietetics in 2002 and her degree as a Certified Nutritionist in 2004, she has helped many clients and workshop attendees to decode their own health dilemmas by understanding the inconsistencies in conventional nutritional dogma. As a cook, her recipes have been popular with everyone from celebrated chefs to picky 4 year olds and adults who "don't eat that". She currently resides in Hawaii with her husband and two children.

She can be found online at http://www.nutritionheretic.com as well as on Facebook (https://www.facebook.com/TheNutritionHeretic) and Twitter(@NutriHeretic).

Made in the USA
Columbia, SC
18 October 2020